Breakthrough to spastic quadriplegic palsy disorder

A step by step guide on how to break stereotypes and embrace practical solutions to spastic quadriplegic palsy

Lily Morgan

Copyright © 2024 by Lily Morgan

Table of Contents

Introduction

Welcome to "How to Overcome Spastic Quadriplegic Palsy: Breaking Stereotypes and Embracing Practical Solutions." This book is a compass for those navigating the complex terrain of spastic quadriplegia, offering insights, inspiration, and tangible strategies for a fulfilling life. Embarking on an exploration of spastic quadriplegia, we unravel its intricacies, providing a foundational understanding of the condition. Moving beyond theoretical insights, we delve into the practical aspects, addressing the daily challenges faced by individuals and introducing adaptive techniques and assistive technologies. Breaking stereotypes is a central theme, challenging preconceived notions through the lens of real-life stories of triumph.

This section aims to reshape societal perceptions, fostering a more inclusive understanding of spastic quadriplegia. Shifting gears towards solutions, we explore holistic approaches to wellness, encompassing physical rehabilitation and strategies for mental and emotional wellbeing. Empowerment takes center stage as we discuss building supportive networks and setting and achieving personal goals. We look ahead to celebrate progress and achievements. This book is not just a guide; it's an invitation to join a journey of empowerment, resilience, and growth. Together, let's challenge stereotypes, embrace practical solutions, and uncover the transformative potential within the realm of spastic quadriplegia.

Chapter 1: Understanding Spastic Quadriplegic Palsy

Spastic Quadriplegic Palsy is a complex neurological condition that profoundly impacts an individual's motor functions and muscle control. This chapter aims to provide a comprehensive understanding of the basics of spastic quadriplegia, offering insights into the nature of the condition and its effects on daily life.

The Basics of Spastic Quadriplegia

At its core, spastic quadriplegia is characterized by a heightened muscle tone, affecting all four limbs and often the trunk. This heightened muscle tone, or spasticity, leads to stiffness and difficulty in voluntary movement. Understanding the biomechanics of spastic quadriplegia is essential in appreciating the challenges individuals face.

Beyond the physical aspects, spastic quadriplegia can impact speech, vision, and cognitive functions, further complicating the overall picture. Recognizing the multifaceted nature of this condition is crucial for anyone seeking to comprehend the experiences of those living with spastic quadriplegia.

Causes and Diagnosis

Exploring the causes of spastic quadriplegia unveils a spectrum of potential factors. While some cases may be linked to genetic factors or prenatal complications, others may result from perinatal or postnatal events. Premature birth, oxygen deprivation, or traumatic brain injuries are among the factors that can contribute to the development of spastic quadriplegia. Diagnosing spastic quadriplegia requires a multidisciplinary approach involving medical professionals, neurologists, and sometimes genetic specialists.

The process often begins with a thorough medical history, followed by a series of physical and neurological examinations. Advanced imaging techniques, such as magnetic resonance imaging (MRI), may be employed to assess the brain's structure and identify any abnormalities. Understanding the causes and diagnostic process not only facilitates early intervention but also plays a crucial role in shaping personalized care plans. This knowledge empowers individuals, families, and healthcare professionals to navigate the challenges associated with spastic quadriplegia more effectively. Grasping the basics of spastic quadriplegia is a foundational step toward fostering empathy and support for individuals living with this condition. By comprehending the causes and diagnostic procedures, we pave the way for early intervention, personalized care, and a more inclusive approach to addressing the complexities of spastic quadriplegic palsy.

Chapter 2: Navigating Physical Barriers

Navigating physical barriers is a significant aspect of living with spastic quadriplegic palsy. This chapter is dedicated to exploring adaptive techniques for daily living and the transformative impact of assistive devices and technologies.

Adaptive Techniques for Daily Living

Living with spastic quadriplegia often requires individuals to develop adaptive techniques that enhance their independence and functionality. These techniques span various aspects of daily life, including personal care, mobility, and communication.

Personal Care: Adaptive techniques for personal care involve finding innovative ways to manage daily hygiene, dressing, and grooming tasks. This may include using specialized tools, adaptive clothing, or modifying daily routines to maximize efficiency while minimizing physical strain.

Mobility: Navigating the physical environment can be challenging, but adaptive techniques can make a substantial difference. Individuals with spastic quadriplegia may explore techniques such as weight-shifting, strategic muscle use, or employing assistive devices like canes or walkers to enhance stability and mobility.

Communication: Adaptive communication techniques are crucial for individuals with spastic quadriplegia, especially if speech is affected.

Augmentative and alternative communication (AAC) methods, such as communication boards, electronic devices, or sign language, empower individuals to express themselves effectively.

By understanding and incorporating these adaptive techniques, individuals can not only overcome physical barriers but also enhance their overall quality of life. It's a continuous process of exploration and adaptation tailored to individual needs and preferences.

Assistive Devices and Technologies

The integration of assistive devices and technologies is a game-changer for those with spastic quadriplegia, providing avenues to overcome physical limitations and participate more fully in various activities.

Mobility Aids: Devices like wheelchairs, scooters, or motorized chairs offer enhanced mobility, enabling individuals to navigate both indoor and outdoor spaces more efficiently. Customized adaptations and accessories further enhance the functionality of these aids.

Orthotic Devices: Orthotic devices, including braces and splints, play a crucial role in providing support and stability to weakened limbs. They are tailored to the individual's specific needs, promoting better posture and minimizing the impact of spasticity on movement.

Communication Devices: Technological advancements have led to a variety of communication devices tailored to individuals with spastic quadriplegia.

Speech-generating devices, eye-tracking technology, and specialized computer interfaces empower individuals to communicate effectively, transcending the limitations imposed by impaired motor functions. **Adaptive Tools for Daily Tasks:** From modified eating utensils to specialized writing tools, adaptive devices for daily tasks empower individuals to engage in activities that might otherwise be challenging. These tools are designed to accommodate varying degrees of motor impairment, promoting independence and participation. The continual evolution of assistive technologies holds immense promise for improving the lives of individuals with spastic quadriplegia.

Integrating these devices and technologies not only breaks down physical barriers but also fosters a sense of autonomy and inclusivity, enabling individuals to actively participate in diverse aspects of life.

This chapter sheds light on the adaptive techniques and assistive devices that form the cornerstone of navigating physical barriers associated with spastic quadriplegic palsy. Through exploration, customization, and integration, individuals can discover a multitude of strategies to enhance their daily experiences and embrace a more fulfilling life.

Chapter 3: Breaking Stereotypes

Chapter 3 delves into the pivotal theme of breaking stereotypes associated with spastic quadriplegic palsy. By addressing common misconceptions and sharing personal stories of triumph, this chapter aims to challenge societal preconceptions and foster a more inclusive understanding of the condition.

Addressing Common Misconceptions

Spastic quadriplegic palsy, like many medical conditions, is often accompanied by prevalent misconceptions rooted in a lack of awareness and understanding. This section is dedicated to dismantling these misconceptions and providing accurate insights into the realities of living with spastic quadriplegia.

One common misconception is the belief that individuals with spastic quadriplegia are intellectually impaired. In reality, the condition primarily affects motor functions, and many individuals with spastic quadriplegia have normal or above-average cognitive abilities. By addressing this misconception, the chapter aims to underscore the importance of recognizing the diversity and individuality of experiences within the spastic quadriplegic community. Another misconception revolves around assumptions regarding the limitations of individuals with spastic quadriplegia. This chapter delves into the varied capabilities and achievements of those with the condition, highlighting that each person's journey is unique and should not be defined solely by physical challenges. By challenging these misconceptions, the narrative shifts from a focus on limitations to one of resilience, potential, and empowerment. Additionally, the chapter confronts stereotypes related to dependency, emphasizing that individuals with spastic quadriplegia can lead independent lives with the right support systems and adaptive strategies. It aims to break down the notion that dependency equates to helplessness, fostering a more accurate and nuanced understanding of the autonomy individuals with spastic quadriplegia can achieve.

Personal Stories of Triumph

Personal narratives have a profound impact on reshaping societal attitudes and breaking down stereotypes. This section shares compelling stories of individuals who have triumphed over the challenges of spastic quadriplegic palsy. These narratives provide a human touch, offering insights into the resilience, strength, and achievements of those living with the condition. Each story highlights unique journeys, shedding light on the diverse ways individuals navigate their lives with spastic quadriplegia.

From educational achievements and career pursuits to personal milestones and community contributions, these narratives serve as powerful examples of the multifaceted capabilities of individuals with spastic quadriplegic palsy. By showcasing these stories, the chapter aims to humanize the condition and challenge preconceived notions. It invites readers to empathize with the experiences of individuals with spastic quadriplegia, fostering a sense of connection and understanding. These stories of triumph not only inspire but also contribute to a broader cultural shift towards inclusivity and acceptance. This part of the book is a call to action against stereotypes associated with spastic quadriplegic palsy. By dismantling misconceptions and sharing personal stories of triumph, this chapter contributes to a more informed, compassionate, and inclusive perspective on the capabilities and potential of individuals living with spastic quadriplegia.

Chapter 4: Holistic Approaches to Wellness

Living with spastic quadriplegic palsy necessitates a comprehensive and holistic approach to wellness. This chapter delves into the multifaceted aspects of well-being, exploring the pivotal roles of physical therapy and rehabilitation, as well as the intricate connections between mental and emotional health.

Physical Therapy and Rehabilitation

Understanding the Importance: Physical therapy and rehabilitation are cornerstones in the holistic care of individuals with spastic quadriplegic palsy. The primary goals are to optimize physical function, enhance mobility, and prevent or manage complications associated with muscle stiffness and impaired motor control.

Customized Treatment Plans: Each individual with spastic quadriplegia presents a unique set of challenges, and thus, a personalized approach to physical therapy is crucial. Skilled physical therapists work collaboratively with individuals, tailoring treatment plans to address specific needs and goals. These plans often incorporate a variety of techniques, exercises, and modalities.

Range of Motion and Strengthening Exercises: Physical therapy aims to improve range of motion and build muscle strength. Therapists design exercises targeting specific muscle groups, employing stretching and strengthening routines to enhance mobility and reduce the impact of spasticity.

Orthotic Interventions: Orthotic devices, such as braces and splints, are frequently utilized in rehabilitation. These aids provide support, stability, and help maintain proper joint alignment, contributing to improved functional abilities.

Gait Training and Mobility Enhancement: For individuals with spastic quadriplegia, gait abnormalities and challenges in mobility are common. Physical therapists engage in gait training, focusing on improving walking patterns and enhancing overall mobility. This includes practicing weight shifting, balance exercises, and utilizing assistive devices when necessary.

Pain Management Strategies: Spasticity often leads to discomfort and pain. Physical therapy addresses pain management through techniques like massage, heat therapy, and specialized exercises aimed at alleviating muscle tension.

In essence, physical therapy and rehabilitation form a dynamic partnership, empowering individuals to navigate their physical capabilities, reduce limitations, and enhance overall quality of life.

Mental and Emotional Wellbeing

Recognizing the Interconnection: The intricate dance between physical health and mental and emotional wellbeing is undeniable. Individuals with spastic quadriplegic palsy navigate not only physical challenges but also grapple with the psychological and emotional aspects of their condition.

Psychosocial Impact: The psychosocial impact of spastic quadriplegia can be profound. Individuals may experience a range of emotions, from frustration and anxiety to grief and resilience. It is crucial to acknowledge and validate these emotions as part of a holistic approach to wellness.

Counseling and Support Services: Mental and emotional wellbeing often benefits from counseling and support services.

Psychologists, counselors, and support groups provide valuable spaces for individuals and their families to express emotions, explore coping mechanisms, and build resilience.

Mindfulness and Relaxation Techniques: Incorporating mindfulness and relaxation techniques into daily routines can significantly contribute to mental and emotional balance. Techniques such as deep breathing, meditation, and mindfulness exercises empower individuals to manage stress, cultivate a positive mindset, and enhance overall emotional resilience.

Quality of Life Enhancement: Fostering mental and emotional wellbeing isn't solely about addressing challenges. It's also about cultivating a sense of purpose, joy, and connection. Engaging in activities that bring fulfillment, setting and achieving personal goals, and maintaining social connections contribute to an enriched quality of life.

Integrated Care Model: Holistic wellness recognizes the interconnectedness of physical, mental, and emotional health. An integrated care model that seamlessly combines medical, rehabilitative, and psychosocial support ensures a comprehensive approach to addressing the diverse needs of individuals with spastic quadriplegia.

In this chapter, we delve into the holistic approaches to wellness essential for individuals living with spastic quadriplegic palsy. From personalized physical therapy interventions that enhance physical function to strategies promoting mental and emotional resilience, this chapter underscores the importance of an integrated approach in fostering overall well-being.

Chapter 5: Empowerment Strategies

Empowerment is at the heart of thriving with spastic quadriplegic palsy. This chapter explores essential empowerment strategies, emphasizing the significance of building a supportive network and the transformative impact of setting and achieving personal goals.

Building a Supportive Network

The Power of Community: Building a supportive network is foundational for individuals with spastic quadriplegic palsy. This network extends beyond medical professionals to encompass family, friends, caregivers, and fellow individuals facing similar challenges. The collective strength of this community provides invaluable emotional, practical, and social support.

Family and Friends: The role of family and friends cannot be overstated. Their understanding, encouragement, and involvement in the individual's life contribute significantly to their overall well-being. Families often play pivotal roles in coordinating care, advocating for resources, and fostering an environment of love and acceptance.

Caregivers and Professionals: Caregivers and healthcare professionals form a critical part of the supportive network. Their expertise in providing physical care, emotional support, and guidance through medical decisions is indispensable. Collaborating with skilled professionals ensures a comprehensive approach to addressing the unique needs associated with spastic quadriplegia.

Peer Support Groups: Connecting with others facing similar challenges can be empowering. Peer support groups provide a platform for individuals to share experiences, exchange practical advice, and find solace in the understanding of shared journeys. These groups foster a sense of belonging and reduce feelings of isolation.

Online Communities: In the digital age, online communities offer avenues for connection and information-sharing. Social media platforms and forums dedicated to spastic quadriplegia enable individuals to access a wealth of knowledge, connect with a global community, and stay updated on advancements in care and technology.

Advocacy Initiatives: Empowerment also involves advocating for broader societal awareness and inclusivity.

Individuals with spastic quadriplegia, along with their support network, can become advocates for accessibility, equal opportunities, and understanding within their communities.

Setting and Achieving Personal Goals

The Power of Goals Setting and achieving personal objectives is a transforming process that promotes empowerment. Goals provide direction, purpose, and a framework for growth. Whether large or little, each completed objective increases an individual's feeling of agency and self-efficacy.

Personalized Goal Planning: Goal setting in the context of spastic quadriplegic palsy requires a personalized approach. Goals may encompass various aspects of life, including physical achievements, educational pursuits, career aspirations, and personal development.

Collaborating with healthcare professionals, rehabilitation specialists, and supportive individuals helps tailor goals to individual abilities and desires.

Incremental Progress: Recognizing the significance of incremental progress is key. Small achievements pave the way for more significant milestones. This approach not only acknowledges the reality of living with spastic quadriplegia but also ensures that each step forward is a celebration of resilience and determination.

Educational and Vocational Goals: Education and vocational pursuits are integral aspects of personal development. Setting goals related to education or career aspirations fosters a sense of purpose and accomplishment. Adaptive strategies and assistive technologies are employed to facilitate active participation in educational and vocational endeavors.

Quality of Life Goals: Goals related to enhancing overall quality of life are equally crucial. These may include social goals, recreational pursuits, and activities that bring joy and fulfillment. Establishing and achieving these goals contribute significantly to an individual's holistic well-being.

This chapter explores empowerment strategies vital for individuals with spastic quadriplegic palsy. Building a supportive network and setting and achieving personal goals are not only integral to navigating the challenges of the condition but also central to fostering a life of purpose, connection, and empowerment.

Conclusion

Throughout the pages of "Breakthrough to Spastic Quadriplegic Palsy: Breaking Stereotypes and Embracing Practical Solutions," the story of spastic quadriplegia emerges as a tapestry woven with tenacity, empowerment, and revolutionary insights. We've looked at the complexities of comprehending the illness, used adaptive ways to overcome physical hurdles, battled preconceptions, embraced holistic wellbeing, and dug into the tactics that enable people to live satisfying lives. This thorough investigation recognizes the varied character of spastic quadriplegic palsy, understanding that people with this illness are defined not by their limits, but by the power of their spirit and the victories they accomplish.

The underlying knowledge presented in the first chapters paved the way for a more informed viewpoint, bridging the gap between awareness and comprehension. Navigating physical hurdles revealed a variety of adaptive solutions, ranging from everyday living tactics to the use of assistive equipment and technology. Breaking preconceptions became a rallying cry, with personal triumphs acting as compelling testaments to the human spirit's tenacity. Holistic approaches to wellness highlighted the connection of physical, mental, and emotional health. The investigation of physical therapy, rehabilitation, and interventions for mental and emotional resilience highlighted the need of a holistic care paradigm in improving overall quality of life.

Empowerment tactics, such as creating a supporting network and establishing personal objectives, emerged key transforming foundations. Families, friends, caregivers, and healthcare professionals worked together to create an atmosphere that promotes empowerment and inclusion. As we get to the conclusion of this book, the story expands beyond the pages of this book to include the life experiences of persons affected by spastic quadriplegic palsy. It is a story about optimism, breaking down boundaries, accepting diversity, and celebrating the victory of the human spirit. May the insights obtained in these chapters spark a larger cultural movement toward understanding, inclusion, and empowerment for those living with spastic quadriplegia.

Consider the enormous influence that will last beyond the pages of this book. The breakthrough is more than just words; it resonates in the hearts and brains of anyone who encounter with these stories. Let this journey serve as a catalyst for societal transformation, inspiring a collective commitment to inclusivity, breaking down barriers, and fostering a future in which individuals affected by spastic quadriplegia are embraced with profound compassion, unwavering support, and a genuine understanding of their extraordinary journeys toward empowerment, resilience, and a life enriched by the triumph of the human spirit.